Healthy Sleep
Happy Kids

A Parents Guide to Sleep Apnea and Kids

For Rahul

Because life without you is unimaginable

HEALTHY SLEEP, HAPPY KIDS

A Parent's Guide to Sleep Apnea and Kids

Published by Soapbox Publishing

First Print Edition, 2018

TABLE OF CONTENTS

CHAPTER 1.

IDENTIFYING SLEEP APNEA

Avery was a typical six year old... or so she thought. But her mom had a different story for us. Avery disliked being woken up for school; she was grumpy and not in a very happy mood all day long. Her grades weren't quite up to what her teachers knew her capabilities were and she often fell asleep during the day. She also suffered from chronic allergies and had dark circles under her eyes.

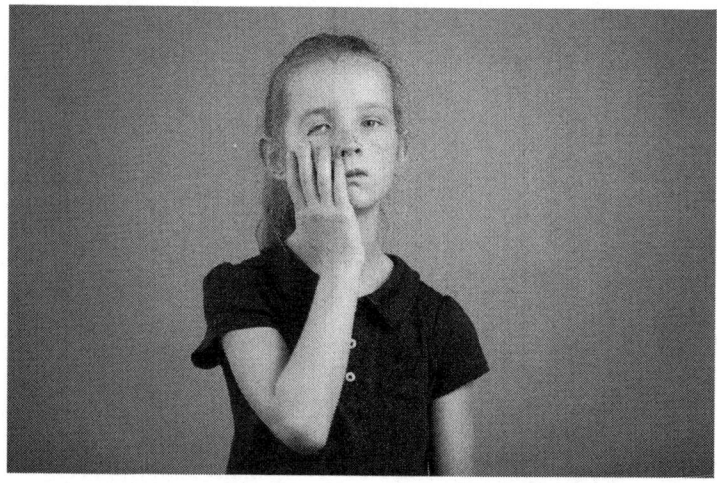

Robby was an active four year old who always had a hard time listening and following directions. He couldn't sit still long enough to focus, and he snored at night. He was also a mouth breather and his mom complained of bad breath no matter how well she brushed and flossed his teeth.

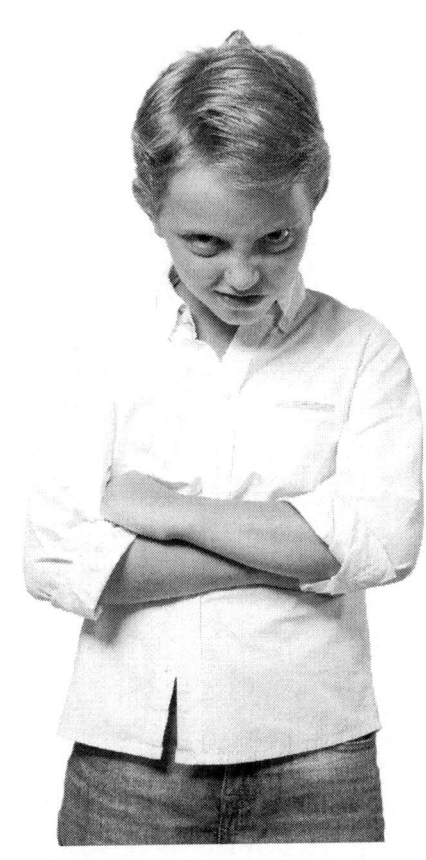

Maddie was a "messy" sleeper and a mouth breather. She suffered from chronic allergies and was always stuffy. She complained of headaches in the morning and was not a "morning person", according to her parents. She made friends easily but was often tired during the day.

Do any of these sound like your child? Do these symptoms resonate with what you see in your kids everyday?

Does your child snore? Does your child show signs of "sleep-disordered breathing": tossing and turning while sleeping, mouth breathing, stopping or pausing breathing while sleeping? These are signs of possible sleep apnea in kids, especially the snoring. This condition is more common than is recognized.

There is a health crisis in our children today and it may or may not be silent. An estimated 9 out of 10 kids suffer from one or more of the following symptoms:

⟹ Tooth grinding

⟹ Heavy breathing while sleeping

⟹ Bedwetting, especially if a child stayed dry previously

⟹ ADD/ADHD

⇒ Snoring

⇒ Daytime sleepiness

⇒ Behavior problems

⇒ Chronic allergies

⇒ Swollen tonsils

⇒ Restless sleep

⇒ Tossing and turning while sleeping

⇒ Nightmares

⇒ Morning headaches

⇒ Depression

Because sleep apnea makes it hard to get a good night's sleep or to feel rested, kids might:

⇒ Have a hard time waking up in the morning

⇒ Be tired during the day

⇒ Have problems focusing at school

⇒ Have behavior problems

As a result, these kids can have poor school performance.

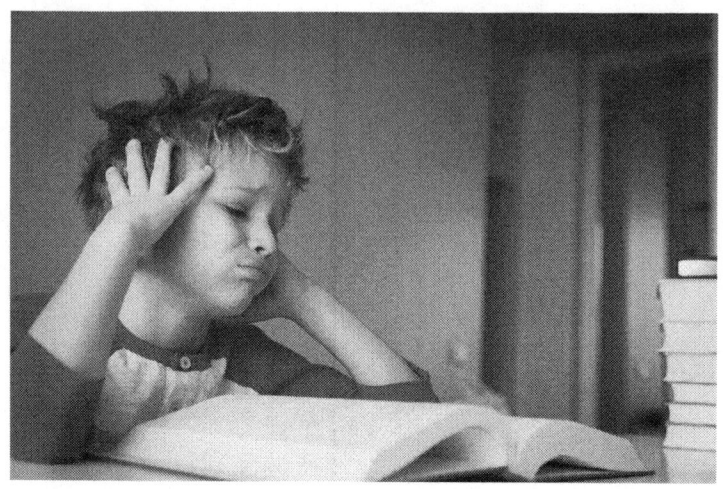

Undiagnosed and untreated sleep apnea contributes to daytime fatigue. Following a night of poor quality sleep, children are more likely to be hyperactive and have difficulty focusing and paying attention.

Teachers and educators can think that such children may have Attention Deficit Hyperactivity Disorder (ADHD) or other learning problems. Recent studies show that kids who snore loudly were twice as likely to have learning problems.

Studies have suggested that about 25% of kids with ADHD may have symptoms of sleep apnea and that their learning and behavior difficulties and problems may be a result of chronic disturbed sleep.

Bedwetting, sleepwalking, slow growth and other hormonal problems can be related to sleep apnea and poor quality of sleep.

Sleep-disordered breathing can and does affect the functions of the brain associated with cognitive capabilities, organization and self-regulation.

The most common treatment options for these cases are usually medications, psychiatric counseling, allergy testing and sometimes sleep studies.

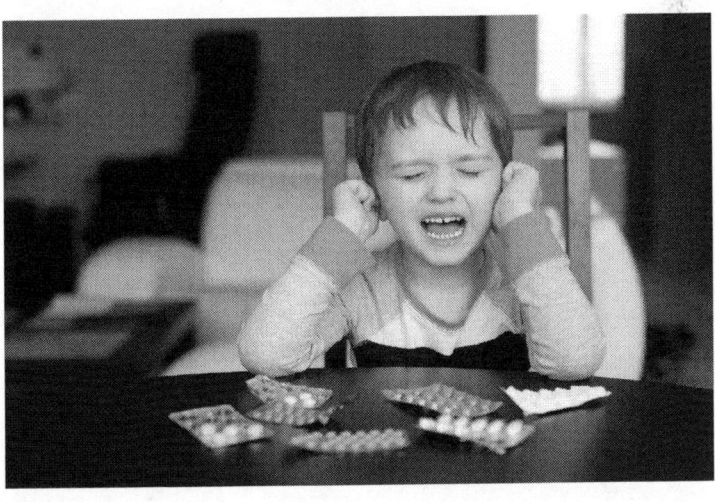

A lot of times these conventional treatment options address only the symptoms, leaving the cause untreated. They act as Band-Aids and have a short lasting effect.

Medications come with unwanted and often plentiful side effects. They can be expensive and time consuming. But there are alternatives, as you will see in a later chapter. But first, the next chapter will cover a closer look at what sleep apnea is.

Chapter 2.

What is Sleep Apnea in Kids?

For a long time, sleep apnea has been regarded as a medical condition only affecting adults. However, the reality is very different, as sleep apnea can also affect kids from infancy to adolescence. Sleep-disordered breathing is common in children. About 3−12% of children have some form of sleep-disordered breathing, which can range from snoring to sleep apnea.

Obstructive sleep apnea occurs when the muscles relax after a child falls asleep. When this happens, the soft tissue at the back of the throat collapses and hinders the flow of air.

Sleep apnea affecting kids may also be a result of oversized tonsils or adenoids which block the airway. This blocking of the airway results in partially reduced breathing called "hypopnea." When there is a complete stoppage in breathing, it is called "apnea."

These obstructions occur throughout the night and disrupt sleep in children. It also results in a lack of sufficient oxygen reaching the brain.

Most of the time, parents ignore the subtle signs and symptoms pointing to sleep apnea in their children. Parents assume that the children will grow out of it. This isn't always the case.

While some children may escape suffering from sleep disorders during growth and development, some children still have to deal with it. When sleep apnea is ignored in kids, it can lead to health problems and can have harmful effects on the child's growth and development.

It is a serious disorder that should not be left untreated as it can lead to medical conditions such as obesity, depression and diabetes in children. Parents and pediatricians consistently need to look out for signs and symptoms that may be pointing to sleep apnea in kids.

Dentists can play a key role in screening for sleep-disordered breathing in kids. Evaluation of the child must include an examination during regular dental checkups along with a detailed questionnaire to be filled out by the parents, which will help guide the dentist in the screening.

We want to make sure that we are not only addressing the symptoms of sleep-disordered breathing in children but also the cause. In the next chapter, you will discover the leading causes of sleep apnea in children.

CHAPTER 3.

CAUSES OF SLEEP APNEA

Various factors contribute to sleep apnea in kids. Common causes start at an early age.

Prolonged use of pacifiers and nipple bottles beyond 6–8 months of age can be a key causative factor by resulting in poor tongue position and swallowing. Prolonged pacifier use hinders proper development of the palate and upper jaw. This leads to lack of adequate space for the tongue. Ideally, the tongue must rest passively in the roof of the mouth and not in the floor of the mouth, as is common belief. Insufficient room for the tongue causes it to fall back into the throat when the child lays down, leading to obstruction. Combined with large tonsils, this can lead to improper breathing and the presence of snoring and insufficient oxygen supply to the brain.

Thumb sucking is another common cause of improper development of the jaws; it also causes mouth breathing and can lead to open bites.

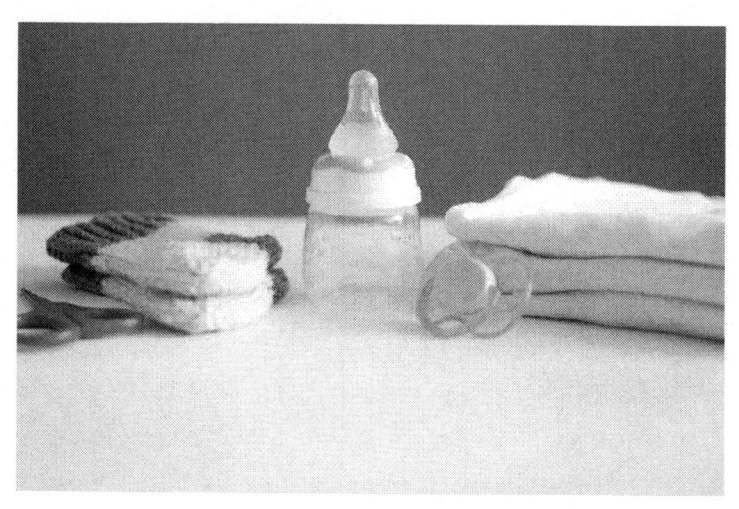

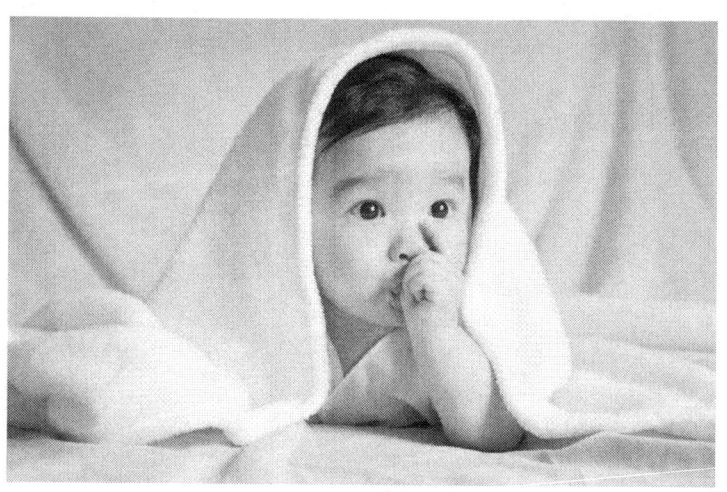

Mouth breathing while sleeping causes airway constriction. This can result in a reduced airway and reduced oxygen uptake by the brain. It affects the neurological, endocrine and hormonal systems, along with immunity.

It results in sleep deprivation symptoms and results in improper mandibular growth.

Some other factors may be quite similar to those causing sleep apnea in adults. More often than not, the main causative factors of sleep apnea in adults are age, neck circumference and weight.

However, in children, enlarged tonsils and/or adenoids can contribute to sleep apnea. These are tissues that fight germs and are located behind the nasal cavity. When these tissues are enlarged in a child, they can cause breathing problems during daytime for kids. When a child having sleep apnea retires to bed, the muscles in the body relax, as well as those in the throat. The relaxation of these muscles, combined with enlarged tonsils and adenoids, can restrict the airflow in the upper respiratory system and lead to sleep apnea.

Obesity can also contribute to sleep apnea in children as it does in adults. There are several studies that show a strong correlation between sleep disorders in kids and childhood obesity. The more fat deposited in the throat muscles, the higher the propensity of sleep apnea occurring in a child. The extra soft fatty tissues result in hindrance to airflow. Usually, obesity can only be suspected as a cause of sleep apnea in older children and not in younger children. Adequate healthy sleep is as important as proper diet and exercise.

Sleep apnea may also be associated with delayed growth in children. Sleep is important in the production of growth hormone, and lack of sleep can contribute to poor growth, along with cardiovascular problems. REM sleep is vital in memory and learning.

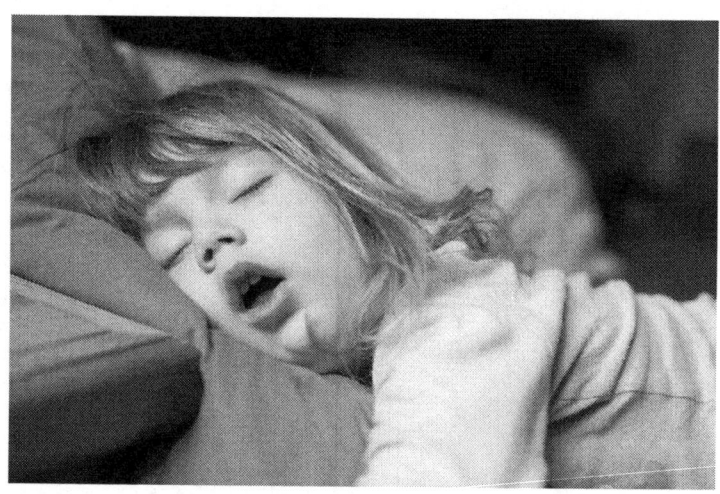

The following risk factors contribute to the development of obstructive sleep apnea in children:

⟹ A hereditary history of obstructive sleep apnea

⟹ A large tongue, which could block the airway during sleep

⟹ "Kissing tonsils" (tonsils that meet or over lap in the middle)

⟹ A defect in the development of oral structures, throat or jaw that may narrow the airway

⟹ Narrow or small-sized arch or jaw

⟹ Prolonged use of pacifier or bottle feeding

⟹ Mouth breathing

⟹ Prolonged habits such a thumb sucking or tongue thrusting

In the next chapter, you will get to know the various signs and symptoms that can help you discover if your child has sleep apnea or not.

Mouth breathing while sleeping causes airway constriction. This can result in a reduced airway and reduced oxygen uptake by the brain. It affects the neurological, endocrine and hormonal systems, along with immunity. It results in sleep deprivation symptoms and results in improper mandibular growth.

Some other factors may be quite similar to those causing sleep apnea in adults. More often than not, the main causative factors of sleep apnea in adults are age, neck circumference and weight.

However, in children, enlarged tonsils and/or adenoids can contribute to sleep apnea. These are tissues that fight germs and are located behind the nasal cavity. When these tissues are enlarged in a child, they can cause breathing problems during daytime for kids. When a child having sleep apnea retires to bed, the muscles in the body relax, as well as those in the throat. The relaxation of these muscles, combined with enlarged tonsils and adenoids, can restrict the airflow in the upper respiratory system and lead to sleep apnea.

Obesity can also contribute to sleep apnea in children as it does in adults. There are several studies that show a strong correlation between sleep disorders in kids and childhood obesity.

The more fat deposited in the throat muscles, the higher the propensity of sleep apnea occurring in a child. The extra soft fatty tissues result in hindrance to airflow. Usually, obesity can only be suspected as a cause of sleep apnea in older children and not in younger children. Adequate healthy sleep is as important as proper diet and exercise.

Sleep apnea may also be associated with delayed growth in children. Sleep is important in the production of growth hormone, and lack of sleep can contribute to poor growth, along with cardiovascular problems. REM sleep is vital in memory and learning.

The following risk factors contribute to the development of obstructive sleep apnea in children:

⟹ A hereditary history of obstructive sleep apnea

⟹ A large tongue, which could block the airway during sleep

⟹ "Kissing tonsils" (tonsils that meet or over lap in the middle)

⟹ A defect in the development of oral structures, throat or jaw that may narrow the airway

⟹ Narrow or small-sized arch or jaw

⟹ Prolonged use of pacifier or bottle feeding

⟹   Mouth breathing

⟹   Prolonged habits such a thumb sucking
        or tongue thrusting

In the next chapter, you will get to know the various signs and symptoms that can help you discover if your child has sleep apnea or not.

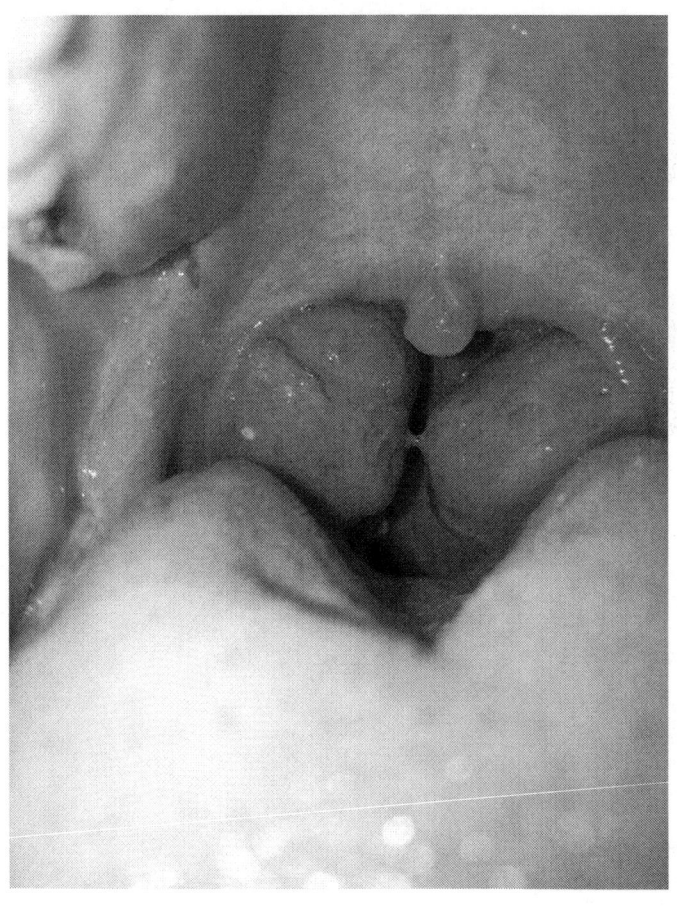

CHAPTER 4.

IDENTIFYING THE SIGNS AND SYMPTOMS OF SLEEP APNEA

When a child with sleep apnea stops breathing, their oxygen level drops. This occurs multiple times a night. These frequent stops result in brief awakenings prompted by the brain so that the airway reopens. This occurs in children without them being aware of these frequent awakenings. Children with sleep apnea experience this cycle of waking and sleeping all through the night. This causes them to be groggy and tired during the day.

Children with obstructive sleep apnea tend to breathe without interruptions during the day, but it has been noted that a number of them breathe through the mouth. These children may experience frequent upper respiratory tract infections. Also, some children have such large tonsils—which are also known as "kissing tonsils"—that it is hard for them to breathe effectively or swallow easily.

The symptoms of sleep apnea in kids tend to appear in the first few years of life. However, the sleep-disordered breathing can often remain undetected for many years after. This condition can affect a child's life in many ways. Such children may experience a delayed growth rate. Generally, behavioral and cognitive issues are noticed more frequently in kids with sleep apnea.

Signs and symptoms of sleep-disordered breathing:

⟹ Short periods of no breathing at all

⟹ Sleeping in odd postures and positions

⟹ Noisy breathing and breathing through the mouth

⟹ Difficulty in paying attention and lack of focus

⟹ Bedwetting

⟹ Cardiovascular problems, e.g. abnormalities or arrhythmia

⟹ General poor performance in school

⟹ Irritability, hyperactivity and occasional aggressiveness

⟹ Morning headache and tiredness

⟹ Poor concentration, lack of retentiveness and behavioral challenges at home and in school

⟹ Excessive sweating at night

⟹ Difficulty in waking up in the morning

⇒ Snoring

⇒ Daytime sleepiness and the general weakness of obese children

⇒ Restless sleep marked by occasional tossing and turning

⇒ ADD/ADHD has been shown to be related to sleep apnea

⇒ Chronic allergies

⇒ Teeth grinding

Children with sleep apnea are more likely to suffer from bedwetting. The current theory behind this is that reduced oxygen probably interferes with the child getting enough REM sleep, which has an effect on the neurological and hormonal systems, which in turn interferes with bladder control.

During the night, a child with sleep apnea may:

⇒ Snore loudly and regularly

⇒ Pause breathing, snort, choke or gasp for breath—even to the point of waking them up and disrupting their sleep

⇒ Sleep restlessly in abnormal positions with their heads in different and unusual positions

⇒ Sweat heavily during sleep

Children suffering from sleep apnea may be too young to or unable to describe their sleeping problems. It is essential for us as parents to observe the general sleeping behavior of our child and make some deductions from it. Getting sleep apnea addressed and treated as soon as it is discovered can save your child from various health challenges that may affect them in the future.

Dentists have the tools and the knowledge to affect development of your child's airway, thus helping them breathe better and allowing the required oxygen to reach their brain. This reduces carbon dioxide buildup in the brain.

Dentists can treat far more than just cavities; they can impact the overall health—and thus the future—of every child.

CHAPTER 5.

DIAGNOSIS OF SLEEP APNEA IN KIDS

Before sleep apnea can be treated, a doctor needs to diagnose this disorder appropriately. Usually, the method used in diagnosis is called a "sleep study". During the sleep study, a variety of body functions such as eye movement, heart rate, brain waves and blood oxygen levels are recorded and monitored during sleep.

The sleep study can help the doctor point to the actual sleep disorder affecting the child. Generally, sleep studies in children are similar to those carried out in adults as they measure nearly all of the same body functions during the study.

Sleep studies can be done at a sleep lab or at home. Those done at home are called HST (home sleep test). These are capable of giving the doctors equally valid and accurate information as a lab sleep test would give. A sleep study done at the lab is also called a "polysomnogram".

During a sleep study, sensors are placed at several spots on the child's body with the aid of tape.

These sensors are connected to a computer to provide vital information while the child is asleep.

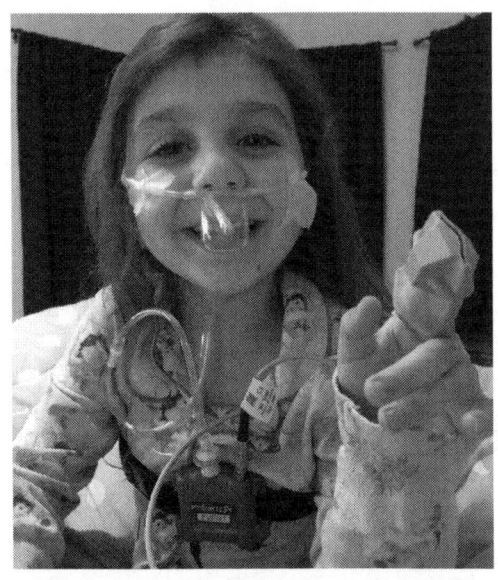

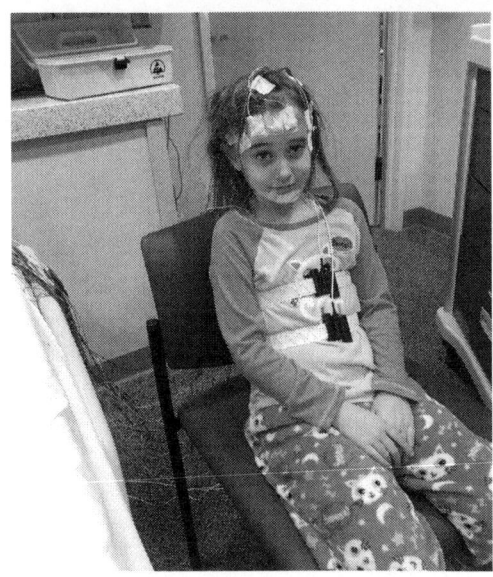

CHAPTER 6.

SUGGESTED TREATMENTS FOR SLEEP APNEA

Untreated sleep apnea in children may result in growth problems and various health issues that may appear later. Treating sleep apnea in children as early as possible can improve their concentration in school, promote emotional stability, improve academic performance and maintain overall wellness.

Children with sleep deprivation and sleep-disordered breathing are generally treated to address their symptoms. However, this tends to be a Band-Aid rather than addressing the root problem. In a growing child, their growth spurts can be used to help the jaws grow desirably to help widen their airway. This chapter will discuss several of these methods and other treatments.

Myofunctional Appliances

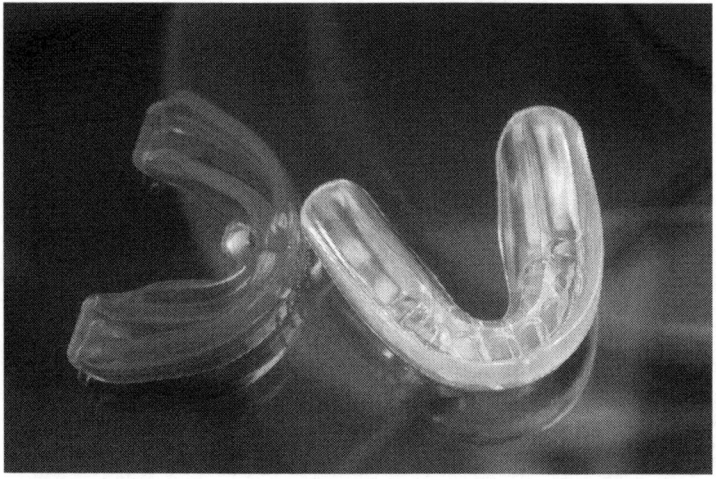

These have been shown to use the child's natural growth patterns and growth spurts to help develop their arch form. They can be implemented in a child as young as two years old. They help address problems such as mouth breathing and are used in habit correction along with tonsil evaluation by the pediatrician or ENT.

Oral myofunctional therapy and appliances can help children retrain their facial and pharyngeal muscles and tongue to return to a more normal pattern of breathing and swallowing.

Myofunctional appliances help in the following ways:

⟹ Expanding the dental arches: The tongue should rest passively in the palate rather than in the floor of the mouth. A well-developed arch leads to a well-developed airway.

⟹ Establishing nasal breathing: Eliminating mouth breathing is a key component in helping increase oxygen intake and delivery to the brain. Breathing through the nose warms and filters the air being sent to the lungs, thus preparing it for optimum uptake.

⟹ Improving other functions: Training the tongue to passively rest in the palate also helps in proper swallowing and speech.

⟹ Eliminating habits such as thumb sucking and tongue thrusting.

Palatal Expanders

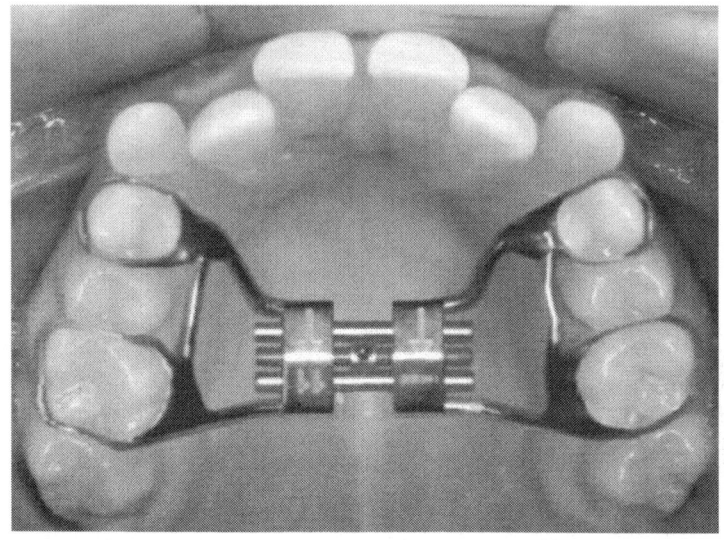

Palatal expanders are fixed to the upper teeth and work to expand the upper jaw in small increments, thus aiding in growth of the airway. Palatal expanders create more space by gradually widening the upper jaw.

During growth, the upper jaw develops as two separate halves that don't fuse together completely until after puberty. Before that time, the two halves can be separated gently and stabilized over a period of several months. Expanding the upper jaw can improve breathing by helping growth of the upper airway.

The expanders can have the benefit of an increase in the nasal airway resistance as well as improved respiratory function.

Daytime-Nighttime Appliances

Daytime-Nighttime Appliances, frequently called DNA appliances, use the patient's own genes to modify and change the position, size and shape of the bone—thus affecting the size and shape of the airway as well. The DNA appliance redirects growth in a way that mimics the development that occurs naturally.

Oral appliances are often an alternative to CPAP to help manage sleep apnea and snoring. DNA appliances bring about a non-surgical remodeling of the upper airway by allowing the body to gently and gradually increase the size of the upper airway and increase the nasal airway as well.

The FDA-approved DNA appliance is worn during the evening and nighttime.

Adenotonsillectomy

This is the most common treatment prescribed for children suffering from sleep apnea. This surgery involves the removal of the adenoids and/or tonsils. This results in a general reduction in the obstruction causing sleep apnea and increases the size of the upper airway. This allows the child to breathe normally during daytime and while sleeping.

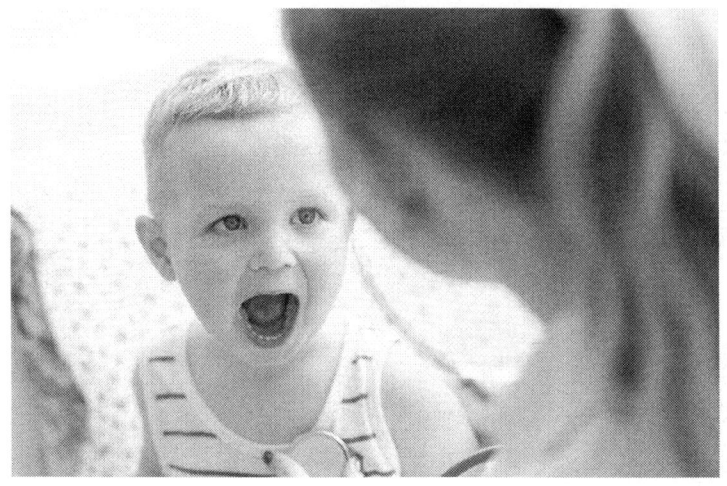

Positive Airway Pressure Therapy

In this treatment, a machine, generally a CPAP, blows air through a tube and mask affixed to the child's nose and/or mouth. The machine used in this procedure sends air pressure to the back of the child's throat to keep it open. This is also the treatment modality with the least compliance. It is considered the gold standard in treatment of sleep apnea but tends to be noisy and cumbersome for a lot of patients.

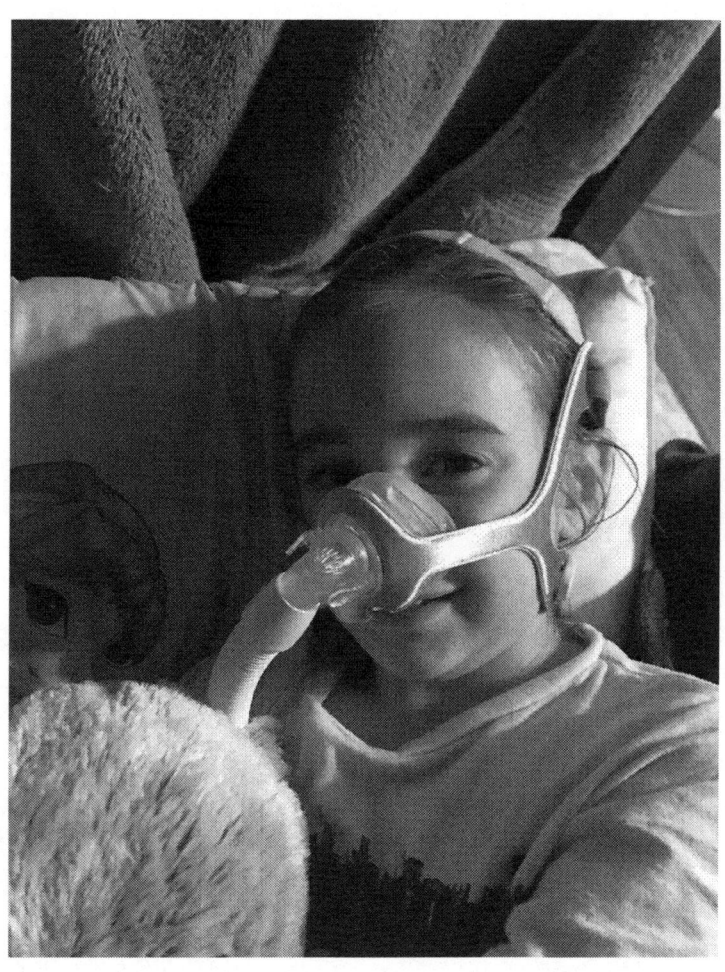

CHAPTER 7.

CONCLUSION

Dentistry today is moving towards a wellness model and the health of our youngest patients is of utmost importance. These kids are our future and dentistry is more than no cavities and straight teeth; we can help our kids BREATHE BETTER!

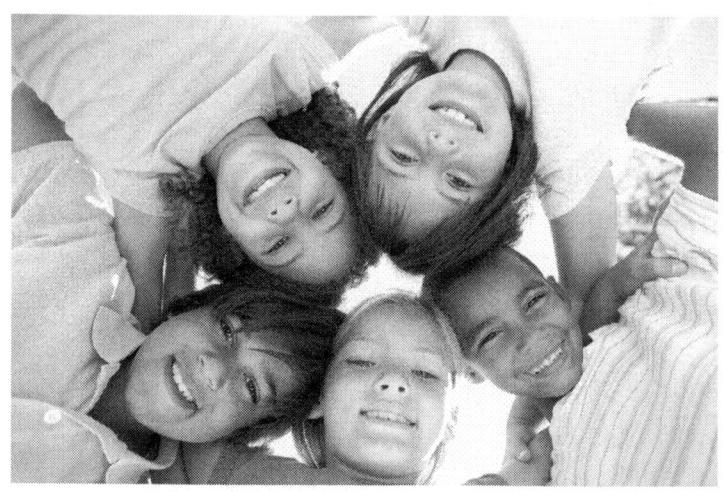

ACKNOWLEDGEMENTS

This would not have been possible without the unwavering love and support of my family. Rahul, who is the wind beneath my wings, my girls, Nandini and Maadhvi, who have been so proud of and amazingly understanding with all my projects. Mom, Dad and Sweta... I love you and miss you guys everyday. My mentor and coach, Dr. Anissa Holmes...Thank you from the bottom of my heart. To my friends, Glenn Vo, Chris Hoffpauir, Paola Bukovcan, Shakila Angadi, Amanda Sheehan, Meghan Darby... you make my heart happy. Last but not least, Christina... my right-hand, my partner in crime, my friend, my shoulder... Thank YOU!!

And a special shoutout to the countless others who have stood by me on this journey. Laura, for your patience with me as I made changes everyday, my team for your encouragement and support. I love you all.

Made in the USA
Lexington, KY
03 April 2019